Make YOUR Life Happen

30 Days to a New YOU!
Diet Companion Workbook/Journal

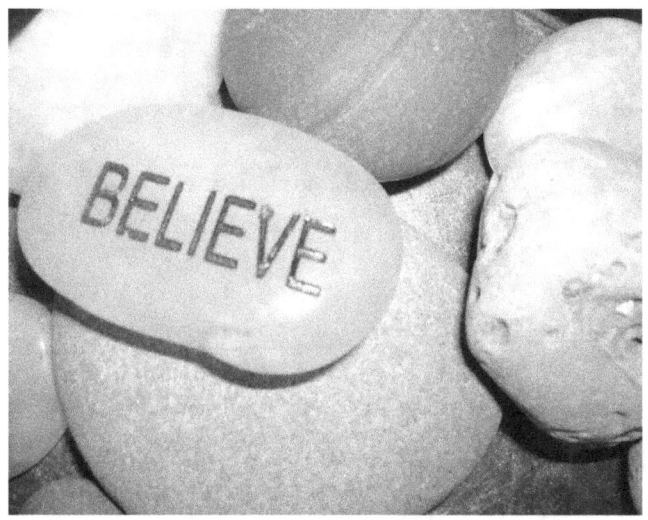

Cristie Will

Cristie Will

Johnstown, CO 80534

www.cbwill.com

www.healthtidings.com

Limits of Liability and Disclaimer of Warranty

The author and publisher shall not be liable for your misuse of this material. This book is strictly for informational and educational purposes.

Warning – Disclaimer

The purpose of this book is to educate and entertain. The author and/or publisher do not guarantee that anyone following these techniques, suggestions, tips, ideas, or strategies will become successful. The author and/or publisher shall have neither liability nor responsibility to anyone with respect to any loss or damage caused, or alleged to be caused, directly or indirectly by the information contained in this book.

Table of Contents

Dedication

I am dedicating this book to everyone that struggles with their weight. My hope is that everyone facing weight issues finds their answer.

Acknowledgements

I want to thank Stephanie Flanders Martin for all your help and insight. Thank you for helping me with a dream of my desires. I have always wanted to walk early in the mornings and I never could do it. Stephanie has given me the help, desire and drive to do just that. Stephanie is a Health and Wellness Coach as well.

I want to thank Maryellen Madden for all her valuable ideas, help, love and continued support. Maryellen is an asset that I am blessed to have.

I want to thank my Daughter, Lauren, for her help getting the word out for our workshops to not only help me, but so that we can help others. I don't have to ask for Lauren's help she just took it upon herself to do these amazing things for me.

Thank you ladies.

Last but not least I want to thank my son-in-law Chris for his help with the workshops as well to get the word out.

Your support and help is priceless.

Introduction

This book is designed to work with any weight loss plan, but particularly with my Books Fat Gone and Connection the Dots to Healthy Weight Loss. This workbook/journal are steps I took and still use to help keep my weight off.

This book is section off by days. Each day has the appropriate pages for Affirmations, Gratitude, Goals and Meal Plan Pages.

This book will start off with some of my favorite quotes. Read these quotes to help give you that extra desire when needed.

Please do your best to do this daily for 30 days and you will see a huge difference in how you feel and look?

I am also including my accelerated boot camp eating plan.

As always consult your Doctor/Physician before starting any exercise and/or diet/weight loss plan.

God Bless and Take Care!

Cristie

DREAMS

Without them the future tastes bland.

"The greatest achievements were at first and for a time dreams. The oak sleeps in the acorn."

~James Allen

All of humanity's amazing accomplishments were once the seeds of someone's dreams.

"Dreams are today's answers to tomorrow's questions."

~*Edgar Cayce*

Someone once dreamed a day might come when they could gaze upon the earth from the vantage point of the moon.

Cristie Will

"Hold fast to dreams, for if dreams die, life is a broken-winged bird that cannot fly."

~Langston Hughes

If we give up on our dreams we give up that which differentiates us from all other creatures—and life becomes condensed to only survival.

"There is only one thing that makes a dream impossible to achieve; the fear of failure."

~Paulo Coelho

Most of what stands in the way of our dreams is us. Dare to get out of your own way.

"Dare to live the life you have dreamed for yourself. Go forward and make your dreams come true."

~Ralph Waldo Emerson

You are the engine that fuels your dreams into reality—your participation is paramount.

"If you can dream it, you can do it. Always remember that this whole thing was started with a dream and a mouse."

~*Walt Disney*

Your mouse is better than Walt's mouse! His didn't even have the internet.

"A dream plus a deadline equals a goal achieved."

~Donna Kozik

If you want your dreams to come true—you have to create a space for them to exist. When you give yourself a deadline you invite your dreams into the real world.

"Whatever you can do, or dream you can, begin it. Boldness has genius, power and magic in it."

~Johann Van Goeth

Your actions propel your dreams into reality.

COURAGE

It's not for the faint of heart.

"It is not because things are difficult that we do not dare; it is because we do not dare that things are difficult."

~Seneca

Courage expressed has a way of changing obstacles into hurdles.

"There is the risk you cannot afford to take, and there is the risk you cannot afford not to take."

~Peter Drucker

Isn't it better to regret the things you *did* than the things you *didn't?*

"Trust that still, small voice that says, "This might work and I'll try it."

~Diane Mariechild

Make friends with that voice. It knows things.

"Courage is not the absence of fear, but rather the judgment that something else is more important than fear."

~Ambrose Redmoon

When your fear of failure is less important than your need to try, courage has a place to breathe.

"Courage doesn't always roar. Sometimes courage is the quiet voice at the end of the day saying, "I will try again tomorrow."

~Mary Anne Radmacher

Spend a few minutes watching a toddler who is learning to walk—that's courage in motion.

"Fear and courage are brothers."

~Proverb

While fear knows nothing of courage, courage knows fear intimately.

"If you have the courage to begin, you have the courage to succeed."

~David Viscott

You don't fall up a mountain. You reach the summit by taking one step after another.

"Life shrinks or expands in proportion to one's courage."

~Anais Nin

Got courage?

FAILURE

The mother of success.

"I have not failed. I've just found 10,000 ways that won't work."

~Thomas Edison

Your perception of the efforts you make on the road to success makes a big difference in the ultimate outcome.

"Fall down seven times. Stand up eight."

~Chinese Proverb

Tap into your inner toddler.

"Failure is an event, never a person."

~William D. Brown

Unsuccessful attempts do not define who you are. Henry Ford failed at his first five business attempts.

"The men who try to do something and fail are infinitely better than those who try to do nothing and succeed."

~Lloyd Jones

The only way to really avoid the possibility of failure—do nothing—also ensures you won't have to deal with success.

"Never confuse a single defeat with a final defeat."

~F. Scott Fitzgerald

Embrace your failures. There is much to learn from them about what doesn't work.

"Failure is the condiment that gives success its flavor."

~Truman Capote

If success was the only possible outcome, what would motivate us to be anything but complacent?

"Only those who dare to fail greatly can ever achieve greatly."

~Robert F. Kennedy

If you wanna be a trapeze artist, you gotta risk falling on your face.

"If we will be quiet and ready enough, we shall find compensation in every disappointment."

~Henry David Thoreau

There is often much more to be learned from our failed attempts at anything than there is from our successes.

PERSPECTIVE

Use it or lose it.

"There is no burnt rice to a hungry person."

~*Philippine Proverb*

Your powers of perception are the most important tools you have to navigate your way through life. Use them wisely.

"We can complain because rose bushes have thorns, or rejoice because thorn bushes have roses."

~Abraham Lincoln

How you see the world directly impacts how the world sees you. If you don't like how you are perceived, change the way you look at things.

"It is a narrow mind which cannot look at subjects from various points of view."

~George Elliot

When you take the time to look at things from many angles you not only expand your awareness, you multiply your opportunities.

"Everything can be taken from a man but one thing: the last of the human freedoms—to choose one's attitude in any given set of circumstances, to choose one's own way."

~Viktor E. Frankl

Attitude and perspective are intertwined. Whether you are mindful of your perspective or not, your attitude will reflect it.

"What we see mainly depends on what we look for."

~John Lubbuck

Challenge yourself to see something or someone differently and watch what happens.

"What you see and hear depends a good deal on where you are standing; it also depends on what sort of person you are."

~C.S. Lewis

No amount of prodding can make a grumpy person congenial. Only they can decide how they see the world.

"Loving people live in a loving world. Hostile people live in a hostile world. Same world."

~Wayne Dyer

Every parent knows a teenager looking for trouble will surely find it. What are you looking for?

"Life is ten percent what you make it and ninety percent how you take it."

~Irving Berlin

It's not really about what shows up in your world as much as it is what you decide to do about it.

"And those who were seen dancing, were thought to be crazy, by those who could not hear the music."

~Friedrich Nietzsche

Your perception of what someone else may be trying to accomplish may not accurately reflect their reality.

EXCUSES

They're rather unbecoming.

"The person who really wants to do something finds a way; the other person finds an excuse."

~Author Unknown

No one really believes the dogs ate the homework anyway—why bother with such silliness?

"Never ruin an apology with an excuse."

~Kimberly Johnson

Sometimes it is better to be excused than to excuse oneself.

"It is better to offer no excuse than a bad one."

~George Washington

If there is no excuse for what you have or haven't done there's no point in compounding the situation.

"It is wise to direct your anger towards problems— not people, to focus your energies on answers—not excuses."

~William Arthur Ward

Every minute spent constructing or elaborating an excuse costs you sixty seconds of solution finding.

"I attribute my success to this: I never gave or took an excuse."

~Florence Nightingale

Never offer an excuse you wouldn't accept.

"If you don't want to do something, one excuse is as good as another."

~Yiddish Proverb

Why waste time making excuses for what you don't want to do instead of making progress with what you do want to do?

"Excuses are the tools with which persons with no purpose in view build for themselves great monuments of nothing."

~Stephen Grayhm

No one makes excuses for getting things done.

"No one ever excused his way to success."

~Dave Del Dotto

You cannot attain excellence in anything by making excuses for mediocre results.

Accelerated Boot Camp Weight Loss Diet

Do's and what you can have:

1. Drink 64 ounces of water a day (Preferably Filtered)
2. Meat, Poultry, Pork and Fish, eggs (Organic) (see Vegan options)*
3. All Vegetables, except Potatoes, Corn and high starch veggies.
4. Blueberries, strawberries, raspberries, and blackberries, lemons, limes, oranges and grapefruit.
5. Healthy fats (Olive, Coconut, Avocado, Nut oils)
6. Nuts (in Moderation unless you are vegan)
7. Balsamic Vinegar and all Vinegar's
8. Take Supplements such as a multi vitamin, Vitamin D3, Red Krill Fish Oil, 5HTP and probiotic.
9. Do the Worksheets every day. Read goals morning and night.
10. Exercise 5 to 6 days a week. Walking is all you have to do.
11. Before going to Bed drink a cup of Dandelion tea. (helps with cleansing out daily toxins)
12. Seasonings are allowed. Salt in moderation.

What you cannot do or have:

1. No processed foods.
2. No Dairy, soy, wheat, corn, sugar, rice or grains.
3. No Corn, Potatoes, or Starchy Vegetables
4. No Pasta, bread, chips, crackers, tortillas
5. No Ice Cream, candy, desserts, or fruit juices

*Vegan/Vegetarian Protein Substitutes, eat more veggies such as:

Broccoli, peas, spinach, kale, sprouts, mushrooms, Brussel sprouts, artichokes, asparagus and really your dark greens in general have more nutrition. Eat more nuts and nut butters. Seeds like sesame, sunflower, hemp and poppy seeds. Add any of these to a smoothie, salads or other vegetables dishes. Eggs is a good source of protein if you eat eggs.

The reason for No Dairy, soy, wheat, corn or sugar is these are the main groups/foods people tend to have allergies to. If you have an allergy to one of these it can hamper your weight loss and it's not good for you. If you really have a craving for one or all these foods you probably are allergic to them or have an intolerance.

At the end of 30 days without dairy, soy, wheat, corn and sugar just add one back into your diet at a time for a few days. You will know if you have an allergy because you will feel terrible. If this is the case quit eating that food and add the next food in and do this until you have re-introduced dairy, soy, wheat, corn and sugar. If you want you can always go and have allergy tests run, this is totally your call.

Example Meal Plan

Breakfast:
Eggs, scrambled, boiled, fried or omelets (choose one)
Bacon, ham, or sausage (choose one)
1 Serving of fruit
Black coffee or tea (no sugar or cream)
Water

Lunch

Salad with olive, coconut oil, nut oils or avocado oil and Vinegar.
Chicken, Pork, beef or fish (one serving)
Roasted Vegetables
Water
Tea or coffee (no sugar or cream)

Snack

Small handful of nuts about 1/4 cup
A few berries

Dinner

Vegetables, baked, roasted, fried or grilled
1 serving of fish, poultry, beef or pork

Water

Do this for the next 30 days and you will have more energy, lose weight and feel better than you have in years that's a guarantee if you follow this plan.

As always consult your Doctor/Physician before starting any exercise/weight loss plan and especially if you have any existing health issues.

If you are on any medications continue to take those as prescribed by your doctor/physician.

I would love to hear from you about your experience on this program. Contact me at www.healthtidings.com.

Affirmations:

I have included my list, but feel free to do your own. Write them daily.

Gratitude

Just journal everyday everything to be thankful for. Examples like someone holding the door open for you, maybe you avoided a wreck, you got a raise or one of your kids did really well in school.

Meal Plan pages

To help you stay on track write down everything you eat and drink. You will be surprised how much you actually consume.

Activity Log pages

The daily activity log is for you to keep track of all activity whether it's vacuuming, walking, running, yoga, strength Training or biking. This will help you see how active you are and help with goals.

Goals

Write goals down daily, even if they have not changed from day one. By writing them down daily it will insure you are checking them daily and reinforcing them day by day.

Day's 1 through 30
Beginning your Transformation

Workbook/Journal

Date:_____

Day 1
To a New YOU!

Goal_____

_____

_____

_____

_____

_____

_____

_____

What Makes your goal
specific?_____

_____

How can your goal be
measured?_____

_____

How is your goal
Attainable?_____

_____

What makes your goal
realistic?_____

_____

What is the timeline for your
goal?_____

_____

DAY #:_____

Meal 1	Portion Sizes	Fat	Calories	Carbs	Protein
TOTALS					
Satisfied after eating?					

Meal 2	Portion Sizes	Fat	Calories	Carbs	Protein
TOTALS					
Satisfied after eating?					

Notes

Meal 3	Portion Sizes	Fat	Calories	Carbs	Protein
TOTALS					
Satisfied after eating?					

Meal 4	Portion Sizes	Fat	Calories	Carbs	Protein
TOTALS					
Satisfied after eating?					

Meal 5	Portion Sizes	Fat	Calories	Carbs	Protein
TOTALS					
Satisfied after eating?					

Daily Activity Log

Date/Time	Activity Description	How I Feel	Duration	Value
NOTES				

Gratitude Journal

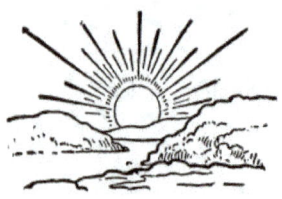

Today's been a Great Day
Because:_____

_____
_____
_____
_____
_____
_____
_____
_____
_____
_____
_____
_____
_____
_____
_____
_____
_____
_____
_____
_____
_____
_____
_____

Example Affirmations you can use or use your own.

Goals:

I choose to set goals, and work to achieve them.

When I set a goal I reach and nothing can stop me.

I stay with my goals until accomplished.

Weight loss:

I live best when I eat less.

I eat only nourishing foods for my Mind, Body and soul.

I feel great at my perfect weight of 120 (fill in the weight you want to weigh)

Self-Esteem:

I love myself more and more every day in every way.

I care about my wellbeing and take care of myself.

I love everything about me.

Exercise:

When I exercise I feel great.

I enjoy exercising

I choose to exercise regularly

Prosperity:

I am a money magnet and money flows freely to me.

Infinite riches are now freely flowing into my life.

It's okay for me to have everything I want.

Health:

I am healthier today and every day.

I choose to be healthy and it shows.

I am vibrantly healthy and radiantly beautiful.

Relationships:

I now give and receive love freely,

I am now attracting my perfect soul mate.

I love to love and be loved.

Happiness:

I feel happy and blissful every day.

Happiness follows me everywhere I go.

I only see and attract happiness.

Affirmations

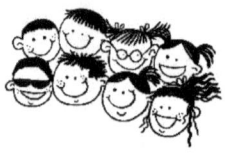

_____! (fill in your own affirmations)

_____

_____

_____

_____

_____

_____

_____

_____

_____

_____

_____

_____

_____

_____

_____

_____

_____

_____

_____

_____

_____

_____

_____

_____

_____

_____

Date:_____

Day 2
To a New YOU!

Goal_____

_____

_____

_____

_____

_____

_____

_____

What Makes your goal
specific?_____

_____

How can your goal be
measured?_____

_____

How is your goal
Attainable?_____

_____

What makes your goal
realistic?_____

_____

What is the timeline for your
goal?_____

_____

DAY #:_____

Meal 1	Portion Sizes	Fat	Calories	Carbs	Protein
TOTALS					
Satisfied after eating?					

Meal 2	Portion Sizes	Fat	Calories	Carbs	Protein
TOTALS					
Satisfied after eating?					

Notes

Meal 3	Portion Sizes	Fat	Calories	Carbs	Protein
TOTALS					
Satisfied after eating?					

Meal 4	Portion Sizes	Fat	Calories	Carbs	Protein
TOTALS					
Satisfied after eating?					

Meal 5	Portion Sizes	Fat	Calories	Carbs	Protein
TOTALS					
Satisfied after eating?					

Daily Activity Log

Date/Time	Activity Description	How I Feel	Duration	Value
NOTES				

Gratitude Journal

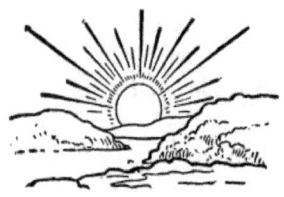

Today's been a Great Day
Because:_____

_____

_____

_____

_____

_____

_____

_____

_____

_____

_____

_____

_____

_____

_____

_____

_____

_____

_____

_____

_____

_____

_____

_____

_____

Example Affirmations you can use or use your own.

Goals:

    I choose to set goals, and work to achieve them.

    When I set a goal I reach and nothing can stop me.

    I stay with my goals until accomplished.

Weight loss:

    I live best when I eat less.

    I eat only nourishing foods for my Mind, Body and soul.

    I feel great at my perfect weight of 120 (fill in the weight you want to weigh)

Self-Esteem:

    I love myself more and more every day in every way.

    I care about my wellbeing and take care of myself.

    I love everything about me.

Exercise:

    When I exercise I feel great.

    I enjoy exercising

    I choose to exercise regularly

Prosperity:

    I am a money magnet and money flows freely to me.

    Infinite riches are now freely flowing into my life.

    Its okay for me to have everything I want.

Health:

    I am healthier today and every day.

    I choose to be healthy and it shows.

    I am vibrantly healthy and radiantly beautiful.

Relationships:

    I now give and receive love freely,

    I am now attracting my perfect soul mate.

    I love to love and be loved.

Happiness:

    I feel happy and blissful every day.

    Happiness follows me everywhere I go.

    I only see and attract happiness.

Affirmations

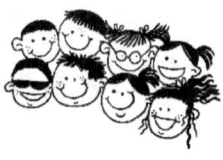

_____! (fill in your own affirmations)

_____
_____
_____
_____
_____
_____
_____
_____
_____
_____
_____
_____
_____
_____
_____
_____
_____
_____
_____
_____
_____
_____
_____
_____

Date:_____

Day 3
To a New YOU!

Goal_____

_____

_____

_____

_____

_____

_____

_____

What Makes your goal
specific?_____

_____

How can your goal be
measured?_____

_____

How is your goal
Attainable?_____

_____

What makes your goal
realistic?_____

_____

What is the timeline for your
goal?_____

_____

DAY #:_____

Meal 1	Portion Sizes	Fat	Calories	Carbs	Protein
TOTALS					
Satisfied after eating?					

Meal 2	Portion Sizes	Fat	Calories	Carbs	Protein
TOTALS					
Satisfied after eating?					

Notes

Meal 3	Portion Sizes	Fat	Calories	Carbs	Protein
TOTALS					
Satisfied after eating?					

Meal 4	Portion Sizes	Fat	Calories	Carbs	Protein
TOTALS					
Satisfied after eating?					

Meal 5	Portion Sizes	Fat	Calories	Carbs	Protein
TOTALS					
Satisfied after eating?					

Daily Activity Log

Date/Time	Activity Description	How I Feel	Duration	Value
NOTES				

Gratitude Journal

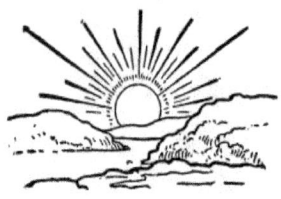

Today's been a Great Day
Because:_____

_____
_____
_____
_____
_____
_____
_____
_____
_____
_____
_____
_____
_____
_____
_____
_____
_____
_____
_____
_____
_____
_____
_____

Example Affirmations you can use or use your own.

Goals:

      I choose to set goals, and work to achieve them.

      When I set a goal I reach and nothing can stop me.

      I stay with my goals until accomplished.

Weight loss:

      I live best when I eat less.

      I eat only nourishing foods for my Mind, Body and soul.

      I feel great at my perfect weight of 120 (fill in the weight you want to weigh)

Self-Esteem:

      I love myself more and more every day in every way.

      I care about my wellbeing and take care of myself.

      I love everything about me.

Exercise:

      When I exercise I feel great.

      I enjoy exercising

      I choose to exercise regularly

Prosperity:

      I am a money magnet and money flows freely to me.

      Infinite riches are now freely flowing into my life.

      It's okay for me to have everything I want.

Health:

      I am healthier today and every day.

      I choose to be healthy and it shows.

      I am vibrantly healthy and radiantly beautiful.

Relationships:

      I now give and receive love freely,

      I am now attracting my perfect soul mate.

      I love to love and be loved.

Happiness:

      I feel happy and blissful every day.

      Happiness follows me everywhere I go.

      I only see and attract happiness.

Affirmations

_____! (fill in your own affirmations)

_____

_____

_____

_____

_____

_____

_____

_____

_____

_____

_____

_____

_____

_____

_____

_____

_____

_____

_____

_____

_____

_____

_____

_____

_____

_____

Date:_____

Day 4
To a New YOU!

Goal_____

_____

_____

_____

_____

_____

_____

_____

What Makes your goal
specific?_____

_____

How can your goal be
measured?_____

_____

How is your goal
Attainable?_____

_____

What makes your goal
realistic?_____

_____

What is the timeline for your
goal?_____

_____

DAY #:_____

Meal 1	Portion Sizes	Fat	Calories	Carbs	Protein
TOTALS					
Satisfied after eating?					

Meal 2	Portion Sizes	Fat	Calories	Carbs	Protein
TOTALS					
Satisfied after eating?					

Notes

Meal 3	Portion Sizes	Fat	Calories	Carbs	Protein
TOTALS					
Satisfied after eating?					

Meal 4	Portion Sizes	Fat	Calories	Carbs	Protein
TOTALS					
Satisfied after eating?					

Meal 5	Portion Sizes	Fat	Calories	Carbs	Protein
TOTALS					
Satisfied after eating?					

Daily Activity Log

Date/Time	Activity Description	How I Feel	Duration	Value
NOTES				

Gratitude Journal

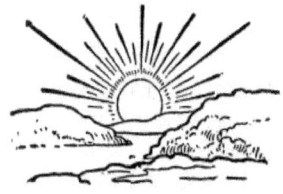

Today's been a Great Day
Because:_____

_____
_____
_____
_____
_____
_____
_____
_____
_____
_____
_____
_____
_____
_____
_____
_____
_____
_____
_____
_____
_____
_____
_____
_____

Example Affirmations you can use or use your own.

Goals:

      I choose to set goals, and work to achieve them.

      When I set a goal I reach and nothing can stop me.

      I stay with my goals until accomplished.

Weight loss:

      I live best when I eat less.

      I eat only nourishing foods for my Mind, Body and soul.

      I feel great at my perfect weight of 120 (fill in the weight you want to weigh)

Self-Esteem:

      I love myself more and more every day in every way.

      I care about my wellbeing and take care of myself.

      I love everything about me.

Exercise:

      When I exercise I feel great.

      I enjoy exercising

      I choose to exercise regularly

Prosperity:

      I am a money magnet and money flows freely to me.

      Infinite riches are now freely flowing into my life.

      It's okay for me to have everything I want.

Health:

      I am healthier today and every day.

      I choose to be healthy and it shows.

      I am vibrantly healthy and radiantly beautiful.

Relationships:

      I now give and receive love freely,

      I am now attracting my perfect soul mate.

      I love to love and be loved.

Happiness:

      I feel happy and blissful every day.

      Happiness follows me everywhere I go.

      I only see and attract happiness.

Affirmations

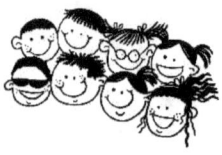

_____! (fill in your own affirmations)

_____

_____

_____

_____

_____

_____

_____

_____

_____

_____

_____

_____

_____

_____

_____

_____

_____

_____

_____

_____

_____

_____

Date:_____

Day 5
To a New YOU!

Goal_____

_____

_____

_____

_____

_____

_____

_____

What Makes your goal
specific?_____

_____

How can your goal be
measured?_____

_____

How is your goal
Attainable?_____

_____

What makes your goal
realistic?_____

_____

What is the timeline for your
goal?_____

_____

DAY #:＿＿＿＿＿

Meal 1	Portion Sizes	Fat	Calories	Carbs	Protein
TOTALS					
Satisfied after eating?					

Meal 2	Portion Sizes	Fat	Calories	Carbs	Protein
TOTALS					
Satisfied after eating?					

Notes

Meal 3	Portion Sizes	Fat	Calories	Carbs	Protein
TOTALS					

Satisfied after eating?	

Meal 4	Portion Sizes	Fat	Calories	Carbs	Protein
TOTALS					

Satisfied after eating?	

Meal 5	Portion Sizes	Fat	Calories	Carbs	Protein
TOTALS					

Satisfied after eating?	

Daily Activity Log

Date/Time	Activity Description	How I Feel	Duration	Value
NOTES				

Gratitude Journal

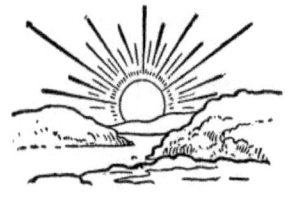

Today's been a Great Day
Because:_____

_____
_____
_____
_____
_____
_____
_____
_____
_____
_____
_____
_____
_____
_____
_____
_____
_____
_____
_____
_____
_____
_____
_____
_____

Example Affirmations you can use or use your own.

Goals:

I choose to set goals, and work to achieve them.

When I set a goal I reach and nothing can stop me.

I stay with my goals until accomplished.

Weight loss:

I live best when I eat less.

I eat only nourishing foods for my Mind, Body and soul.

I feel great at my perfect weight of 120 (fill in the weight you want to weigh)

Self-Esteem:

I love myself more and more every day in every way.

I care about my wellbeing and take care of myself.

I love everything about me.

Exercise:

When I exercise I feel great.

I enjoy exercising

I choose to exercise regularly

Prosperity:

I am a money magnet and money flows freely to me.

Infinite riches are now freely flowing into my life.

It's okay for me to have everything I want.

Health:

I am healthier today and every day.

I choose to be healthy and it shows.

I am vibrantly healthy and radiantly beautiful.

Relationships:

I now give and receive love freely,

I am now attracting my perfect soul mate.

I love to love and be loved.

Happiness:

I feel happy and blissful every day.

Happiness follows me everywhere I go.

I only see and attract happiness.

Affirmations

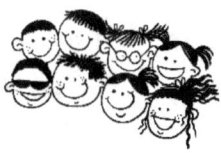

_____! (fill in your own affirmations)

_____
_____
_____
_____
_____
_____
_____
_____
_____
_____
_____
_____
_____
_____
_____
_____
_____
_____
_____
_____
_____
_____
_____
_____
_____
_____

Date:_____

Day 6
To a New YOU!

Goal_____

_____

_____

_____

_____

_____

_____

_____

What Makes your goal
specific?_____
_____

How can your goal be
measured?_____
_____

How is your goal
Attainable?_____
_____

What makes your goal
realistic?_____
_____

What is the timeline for your
goal?_____
_____

DAY #:_____

Meal 1	Portion Sizes	Fat	Calories	Carbs	Protein
TOTALS					
Satisfied after eating?					

Meal 2	Portion Sizes	Fat	Calories	Carbs	Protein
TOTALS					
Satisfied after eating?					

Notes

Meal 3	Portion Sizes	Fat	Calories	Carbs	Protein
TOTALS					
Satisfied after eating?					

Meal 4	Portion Sizes	Fat	Calories	Carbs	Protein
TOTALS					
Satisfied after eating?					

Meal 5	Portion Sizes	Fat	Calories	Carbs	Protein
TOTALS					
Satisfied after eating?					

Daily Activity Log

Date/Time	Activity Description	How I Feel	Duration	Value
NOTES				

Gratitude Journal

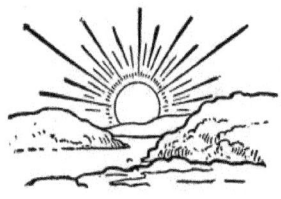

Today's been a Great Day
Because:_____

_____
_____
_____
_____
_____
_____
_____
_____
_____
_____
_____
_____
_____
_____
_____
_____
_____
_____
_____
_____
_____
_____
_____

Example Affirmations you can use or use your own.

Goals:
> I choose to set goals, and work to achieve them.
> When I set a goal I reach and nothing can stop me.
> I stay with my goals until accomplished.

Weight loss:
> I live best when I eat less.
> I eat only nourishing foods for my Mind, Body and soul.
> I feel great at my perfect weight of 120 (fill in the weight you want to weigh)

Self-Esteem:
> I love myself more and more every day in every way.
> I care about my wellbeing and take care of myself.
> I love everything about me.

Exercise:
> When I exercise I feel great.
> I enjoy exercising
> I choose to exercise regularly

Prosperity:
> I am a money magnet and money flows freely to me.
> Infinite riches are now freely flowing into my life.
> It's okay for me to have everything I want.

Health:
> I am healthier today and every day.
> I choose to be healthy and it shows.
> I am vibrantly healthy and radiantly beautiful.

Relationships:
> I now give and receive love freely,
> I am now attracting my perfect soul mate.
> I love to love and be loved.

Happiness:
> I feel happy and blissful every day.
> Happiness follows me everywhere I go.
> I only see and attract happiness.

Affirmations

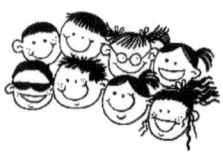

_____! (fill in your own affirmations)

_____

_____

_____

_____

_____

_____

_____

_____

_____

_____

_____

_____

_____

_____

_____

_____

_____

_____

_____

_____

_____

_____

Date:_____

Day 7
To a New YOU!

Goal_____

_____

_____

_____

_____

_____

_____

_____

What Makes your goal
specific?_____

_____

How can your goal be
measured?_____

_____

How is your goal
Attainable?_____

_____

What makes your goal
realistic?_____

_____

What is the timeline for your
goal?_____

_____

DAY #:_____

Meal 1	Portion Sizes	Fat	Calories	Carbs	Protein
TOTALS					
Satisfied after eating?					

Meal 2	Portion Sizes	Fat	Calories	Carbs	Protein
TOTALS					
Satisfied after eating?					

Notes

Meal 3	Portion Sizes	Fat	Calories	Carbs	Protein
TOTALS					
Satisfied after eating?					

Meal 4	Portion Sizes	Fat	Calories	Carbs	Protein
TOTALS					
Satisfied after eating?					

Meal 5	Portion Sizes	Fat	Calories	Carbs	Protein
TOTALS					
Satisfied after eating?					

Daily Activity Log

Date/Time	Activity Description	How I Feel	Duration	Value
NOTES				

Gratitude Journal

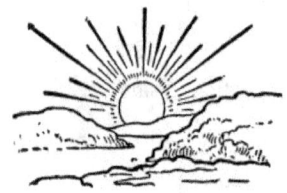

Today's been a Great Day
Because:_____

_____

_____

_____

_____

_____

_____

_____

_____

_____

_____

_____

_____

_____

_____

_____

_____

_____

_____

_____

_____

_____

_____

_____

Example Affirmations you can use or use your own.

Goals:
>   I choose to set goals, and work to achieve them.
>   When I set a goal I reach and nothing can stop me.
>   I stay with my goals until accomplished.

Weight loss:
>   I live best when I eat less.
>   I eat only nourishing foods for my Mind, Body and soul.
>   I feel great at my perfect weight of 120 (fill in the weight you want to
weigh)

Self-Esteem:
>   I love myself more and more every day in every way.
>   I care about my wellbeing and take care of myself.
>   I love everything about me.

Exercise:
>   When I exercise I feel great.
>   I enjoy exercising
>   I choose to exercise regularly

Prosperity:
>   I am a money magnet and money flows freely to me.
>   Infinite riches are now freely flowing into my life.
>   It's okay for me to have everything I want.

Health:
>   I am healthier today and every day.
>   I choose to be healthy and it shows.
>   I am vibrantly healthy and radiantly beautiful.

Relationships:
>   I now give and receive love freely,
>   I am now attracting my perfect soul mate.
>   I love to love and be loved.

Happiness:
>   I feel happy and blissful every day.
>   Happiness follows me everywhere I go.
>   I only see and attract happiness.

Affirmations

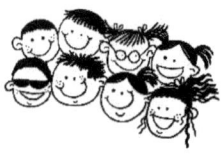

_____! (fill in your own affirmations)

_____

_____

_____

_____

_____

_____

_____

_____

_____

_____

_____

_____

_____

_____

_____

_____

_____

_____

_____

_____

_____

_____

_____

_____

_____

_____

_____

Date:_____

Day 8
To a New YOU!

Goal_____

_____

_____

_____

_____

_____

_____

_____

What Makes your goal
specific?_____

_____

How can your goal be
measured?_____

_____

How is your goal
Attainable?_____

_____

What makes your goal
realistic?_____

_____

What is the timeline for your
goal?_____

_____

DAY #:_____

Meal 1	Portion Sizes	Fat	Calories	Carbs	Protein
TOTALS					
Satisfied after eating?					

Meal 2	Portion Sizes	Fat	Calories	Carbs	Protein
TOTALS					
Satisfied after eating?					

Notes

Meal 3	Portion Sizes	Fat	Calories	Carbs	Protein
TOTALS					
Satisfied after eating?					

Meal 4	Portion Sizes	Fat	Calories	Carbs	Protein
TOTALS					
Satisfied after eating?					

Meal 5	Portion Sizes	Fat	Calories	Carbs	Protein
TOTALS					
Satisfied after eating?					

Daily Activity Log

Date/Time	Activity Description	How I Feel	Duration	Value
NOTES				

Gratitude Journal

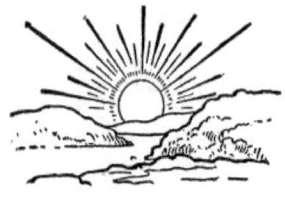

Today's been a Great Day
Because:_____

_____

_____

_____

_____

_____

_____

_____

_____

_____

_____

_____

_____

_____

_____

_____

_____

_____

_____

_____

_____

_____

_____

_____

_____

_____

Example Affirmations you can use or use your own.

Goals:

        I choose to set goals, and work to achieve them.

        When I set a goal I reach and nothing can stop me.

        I stay with my goals until accomplished.

Weight loss:

        I live best when I eat less.

        I eat only nourishing foods for my Mind, Body and soul.

        I feel great at my perfect weight of 120 (fill in the weight you want to weigh)

Self-Esteem:

        I love myself more and more every day in every way.

        I care about my wellbeing and take care of myself.

        I love everything about me.

Exercise:

        When I exercise I feel great.

        I enjoy exercising

        I choose to exercise regularly

Prosperity:

        I am a money magnet and money flows freely to me.

        Infinite riches are now freely flowing into my life.

        It's okay for me to have everything I want.

Health:

        I am healthier today and every day.

        I choose to be healthy and it shows.

        I am vibrantly healthy and radiantly beautiful.

Relationships:

        I now give and receive love freely,

        I am now attracting my perfect soul mate.

        I love to love and be loved.

Happiness:

        I feel happy and blissful every day.

        Happiness follows me everywhere I go.

        I only see and attract happiness.

Affirmations

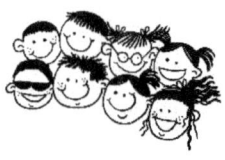

_____! (fill in your own affirmations)

_____

_____

_____

_____

_____

_____

_____

_____

_____

_____

_____

_____

_____

_____

_____

_____

_____

_____

_____

_____

_____

Date:_____

Day 9
To a New YOU!

Goal_____

_____

_____

_____

_____

_____

_____

_____

_____

What Makes your goal
specific?_____

_____

How can your goal be
measured?_____

_____

How is your goal
Attainable?_____

_____

What makes your goal
realistic?_____

_____

What is the timeline for your
goal?_____

_____

DAY #:_____

Meal 1	Portion Sizes	Fat	Calories	Carbs	Protein
TOTALS					
Satisfied after eating?					

Meal 2	Portion Sizes	Fat	Calories	Carbs	Protein
TOTALS					
Satisfied after eating?					

Notes

Meal 3	Portion Sizes	Fat	Calories	Carbs	Protein
TOTALS					
Satisfied after eating?					

Meal 4	Portion Sizes	Fat	Calories	Carbs	Protein
TOTALS					
Satisfied after eating?					

Meal 5	Portion Sizes	Fat	Calories	Carbs	Protein
TOTALS					
Satisfied after eating?					

Daily Activity Log

Date/Time	Activity Description	How I Feel	Duration	Value
NOTES				

Gratitude Journal

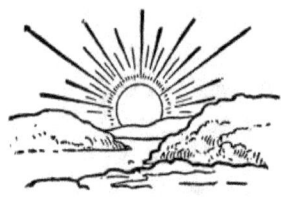

Today's been a Great Day
Because:_____

_____
_____
_____
_____
_____
_____
_____
_____
_____
_____
_____
_____
_____
_____
_____
_____
_____
_____
_____
_____
_____
_____
_____
_____
_____
_____

Example Affirmations you can use or use your own.

Goals:
> I choose to set goals, and work to achieve them.
> When I set a goal I reach and nothing can stop me.
> I stay with my goals until accomplished.

Weight loss:
> I live best when I eat less.
> I eat only nourishing foods for my Mind, Body and soul.
> I feel great at my perfect weight of 120 (fill in the weight you want to weigh)

Self-Esteem:
> I love myself more and more every day in every way.
> I care about my wellbeing and take care of myself.
> I love everything about me.

Exercise:
> When I exercise I feel great.
> I enjoy exercising
> I choose to exercise regularly

Prosperity:
> I am a money magnet and money flows freely to me.
> Infinite riches are now freely flowing into my life.
> It's okay for me to have everything I want.

Health:
> I am healthier today and every day.
> I choose to be healthy and it shows.
> I am vibrantly healthy and radiantly beautiful.

Relationships:
> I now give and receive love freely,
> I am now attracting my perfect soul mate.
> I love to love and be loved.

Happiness:
> I feel happy and blissful every day.
> Happiness follows me everywhere I go.
> I only see and attract happiness.

Affirmations

_____! (fill in your own affirmations)

_____

_____

_____

_____

_____

_____

_____

_____

_____

_____

_____

_____

_____

_____

_____

_____

_____

_____

_____

_____

_____

_____

_____

Date:_____

Day 10
To a New YOU!

Goal_____

_____

_____

_____

_____

_____

_____

_____

What Makes your goal
specific?_____

_____

How can your goal be
measured?_____

_____

How is your goal
Attainable?_____

_____

What makes your goal
realistic?_____

_____

What is the timeline for your
goal?_____

_____

DAY #:_____

Meal 1	Portion Sizes	Fat	Calories	Carbs	Protein
TOTALS					
Satisfied after eating?					

Meal 2	Portion Sizes	Fat	Calories	Carbs	Protein
TOTALS					
Satisfied after eating?					

Notes

Meal 3	Portion Sizes	Fat	Calories	Carbs	Protein
TOTALS					
Satisfied after eating?					

Meal 4	Portion Sizes	Fat	Calories	Carbs	Protein
TOTALS					
Satisfied after eating?					

Meal 5	Portion Sizes	Fat	Calories	Carbs	Protein
TOTALS					
Satisfied after eating?					

Daily Activity Log

Date/Time	Activity Description	How I Feel	Duration	Value
NOTES				

Gratitude Journal

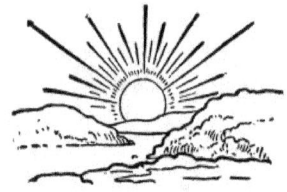

Today's been a Great Day
Because:_____

_____
_____
_____
_____
_____
_____
_____
_____
_____
_____
_____
_____
_____
_____
_____
_____
_____
_____
_____
_____
_____
_____
_____
_____

Example Affirmations you can use or use your own.

Goals:
> I choose to set goals, and work to achieve them.
> When I set a goal I reach and nothing can stop me.
> I stay with my goals until accomplished.

Weight loss:
> I live best when I eat less.
> I eat only nourishing foods for my Mind, Body and soul.
> I feel great at my perfect weight of 120 (fill in the weight you want to weigh)

Self-Esteem:
> I love myself more and more every day in every way.
> I care about my wellbeing and take care of myself.
> I love everything about me.

Exercise:
> When I exercise I feel great.
> I enjoy exercising
> I choose to exercise regularly

Prosperity:
> I am a money magnet and money flows freely to me.
> Infinite riches are now freely flowing into my life.
> It's okay for me to have everything I want.

Health:
> I am healthier today and every day.
> I choose to be healthy and it shows.
> I am vibrantly healthy and radiantly beautiful.

Relationships:
> I now give and receive love freely,
> I am now attracting my perfect soul mate.
> I love to love and be loved.

Happiness:
> I feel happy and blissful every day.
> Happiness follows me everywhere I go.
> I only see and attract happiness.

Affirmations

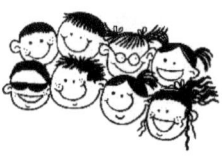

_____! (fill in your own affirmations)

_____

_____

_____

_____

_____

_____

_____

_____

_____

_____

_____

_____

_____

_____

_____

_____

_____

_____

_____

_____

_____

_____

_____

_____

_____

_____

_____

_____

Date:_____

Day 11
To a New YOU!

Goal_____

_____

_____

_____

_____

_____

_____

_____

What Makes your goal
specific?_____

_____

How can your goal be
measured?_____

_____

How is your goal
Attainable?_____

_____

What makes your goal
realistic?_____

_____

What is the timeline for your
goal?_____

_____

DAY #:_____

Meal 1	Portion Sizes	Fat	Calories	Carbs	Protein
TOTALS					
Satisfied after eating?					
Meal 2	Portion Sizes	Fat	Calories	Carbs	Protein
TOTALS					
Satisfied after eating?					

Notes

Meal 3	Portion Sizes	Fat	Calories	Carbs	Protein
TOTALS					
Satisfied after eating?					

Meal 4	Portion Sizes	Fat	Calories	Carbs	Protein
TOTALS					
Satisfied after eating?					

Meal 5	Portion Sizes	Fat	Calories	Carbs	Protein
TOTALS					
Satisfied after eating?					

Daily Activity Log

Date/Time	Activity Description	How I Feel	Duration	Value
NOTES				

Gratitude Journal

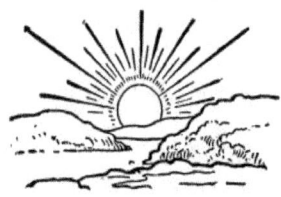

Today's been a Great Day
Because:_____

_____
_____
_____
_____
_____
_____
_____
_____
_____
_____
_____
_____
_____
_____
_____
_____
_____
_____
_____
_____
_____
_____
_____

Example Affirmations you can use or use your own.

Goals:

      I choose to set goals, and work to achieve them.

      When I set a goal I reach and nothing can stop me.

      I stay with my goals until accomplished.

Weight loss:

      I live best when I eat less.

      I eat only nourishing foods for my Mind, Body and soul.

      I feel great at my perfect weight of 120 (fill in the weight you want to weigh)

Self-Esteem:

      I love myself more and more every day in every way.

      I care about my wellbeing and take care of myself.

      I love everything about me.

Exercise:

      When I exercise I feel great.

      I enjoy exercising

      I choose to exercise regularly

Prosperity:

      I am a money magnet and money flows freely to me.

      Infinite riches are now freely flowing into my life.

      It's okay for me to have everything I want.

Health:

      I am healthier today and every day.

      I choose to be healthy and it shows.

      I am vibrantly healthy and radiantly beautiful.

Relationships:

      I now give and receive love freely,

      I am now attracting my perfect soul mate.

      I love to love and be loved.

Happiness:

      I feel happy and blissful every day.

      Happiness follows me everywhere I go.

      I only see and attract happiness.

Affirmations

_____! (fill in your own affirmations)

_____

_____

_____

_____

_____

_____

_____

_____

_____

_____

_____

_____

_____

_____

_____

_____

_____

_____

_____

_____

_____

_____

_____

_____

Date:_____

Day 12
To a New YOU!

Goal_____

_____

_____

_____

_____

_____

_____

_____

What Makes your goal
specific?_____

_____

How can your goal be
measured?_____

_____

How is your goal
Attainable?_____

_____

What makes your goal
realistic?_____

_____

What is the timeline for your
goal?_____

_____

Date:_____

Day 12
To a New YOU!

Goal_____

_____

_____

_____

_____

_____

_____

_____

_____

What Makes your goal
specific?_____

_____

How can your goal be
measured?_____

_____

How is your goal
Attainable?_____

_____

What makes your goal
realistic?_____

_____

What is the timeline for your
goal?_____

_____

DAY #:_____

Meal 1	Portion Sizes	Fat	Calories	Carbs	Protein
TOTALS					
Satisfied after eating?					

Meal 2	Portion Sizes	Fat	Calories	Carbs	Protein
TOTALS					
Satisfied after eating?					

Notes

Meal 3	Portion Sizes	Fat	Calories	Carbs	Protein
TOTALS					
Satisfied after eating?					

Meal 4	Portion Sizes	Fat	Calories	Carbs	Protein
TOTALS					
Satisfied after eating?					

Meal 5	Portion Sizes	Fat	Calories	Carbs	Protein
TOTALS					
Satisfied after eating?					

Daily Activity Log

Date/Time	Activity Description	How I Feel	Duration	Value
NOTES				

Gratitude Journal

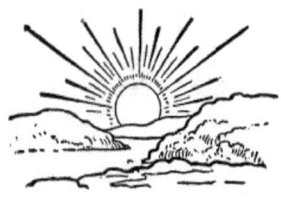

Today's been a Great Day
Because:_____

_____
_____
_____
_____
_____
_____
_____
_____
_____
_____
_____
_____
_____
_____
_____
_____
_____
_____
_____
_____
_____
_____
_____

Example Affirmations you can use or use your own.

Goals:

> I choose to set goals, and work to achieve them.
> When I set a goal I reach and nothing can stop me.
> I stay with my goals until accomplished.

Weight loss:

> I live best when I eat less.
> I eat only nourishing foods for my Mind, Body and soul.
> I feel great at my perfect weight of 120 (fill in the weight you want to weigh)

Self-Esteem:

> I love myself more and more every day in every way.
> I care about my wellbeing and take care of myself.
> I love everything about me.

Exercise:

> When I exercise I feel great.
> I enjoy exercising
> I choose to exercise regularly

Prosperity:

> I am a money magnet and money flows freely to me.
> Infinite riches are now freely flowing into my life.
> It's okay for me to have everything I want.

Health:

> I am healthier today and every day.
> I choose to be healthy and it shows.
> I am vibrantly healthy and radiantly beautiful.

Relationships:

> I now give and receive love freely,
> I am now attracting my perfect soul mate.
> I love to love and be loved.

Happiness:

> I feel happy and blissful every day.
> Happiness follows me everywhere I go.
> I only see and attract happiness.

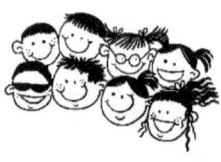

Affirmations

_____! (fill in your own affirmations)

_____

_____

_____

_____

_____

_____

_____

_____

_____

_____

_____

_____

_____

_____

_____

_____

_____

_____

_____

_____

_____

_____

_____

_____

Date:_____

Day 13
To a New YOU!

Goal_____

_____

_____

_____

_____

_____

_____

_____

What Makes your goal
specific?_____

_____

How can your goal be
measured?_____

_____

How is your goal
Attainable?_____

_____

What makes your goal
realistic?_____

_____

What is the timeline for your
goal?_____

_____

DAY #:_____

Meal 1	Portion Sizes	Fat	Calories	Carbs	Protein
TOTALS					
Satisfied after eating?					

Meal 2	Portion Sizes	Fat	Calories	Carbs	Protein
TOTALS					
Satisfied after eating?					

Notes

Meal 3	Portion Sizes	Fat	Calories	Carbs	Protein
TOTALS					

Satisfied after eating? (..............)

Meal 4	Portion Sizes	Fat	Calories	Carbs	Protein
TOTALS					

Satisfied after eating? (..............)

Meal 5	Portion Sizes	Fat	Calories	Carbs	Protein
TOTALS					

Satisfied after eating? (..............)

Daily Activity Log

Date/Time	Activity Description	How I Feel	Duration	Value
NOTES				

Gratitude Journal

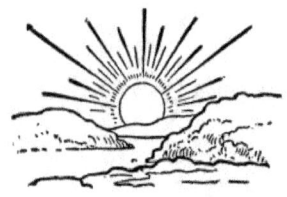

Today's been a Great Day
Because:_____

_____
_____
_____
_____
_____
_____
_____
_____
_____
_____
_____
_____
_____
_____
_____
_____
_____
_____
_____
_____
_____
_____
_____
_____

Example Affirmations you can use or use your own.

Goals:
> I choose to set goals, and work to achieve them.
> When I set a goal I reach and nothing can stop me.
> I stay with my goals until accomplished.

Weight loss:
> I live best when I eat less.
> I eat only nourishing foods for my Mind, Body and soul.
> I feel great at my perfect weight of 120 (fill in the weight you want to weigh)

Self-Esteem:
> I love myself more and more every day in every way.
> I care about my wellbeing and take care of myself.
> I love everything about me.

Exercise:
> When I exercise I feel great.
> I enjoy exercising
> I choose to exercise regularly

Prosperity:
> I am a money magnet and money flows freely to me.
> Infinite riches are now freely flowing into my life.
> It's okay for me to have everything I want.

Health:
> I am healthier today and every day.
> I choose to be healthy and it shows.
> I am vibrantly healthy and radiantly beautiful.

Relationships:
> I now give and receive love freely,
> I am now attracting my perfect soul mate.
> I love to love and be loved.

Happiness:
> I feel happy and blissful every day.
> Happiness follows me everywhere I go.
> I only see and attract happiness.

Affirmations

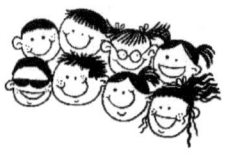

_____! (fill in your own affirmations)

_____

_____

_____

_____

_____

_____

_____

_____

_____

_____

_____

_____

_____

_____

_____

_____

_____

_____

_____

_____

_____

_____

_____

Date:_____

Day 14
To a New YOU!

Goal_____

_____

_____

_____

_____

_____

_____

_____

What Makes your goal
specific?_____

_____

How can your goal be
measured?_____

_____

How is your goal
Attainable?_____

_____

What makes your goal
realistic?_____

_____

What is the timeline for your
goal?_____

_____

DAY #:_____

Meal 1		Portion Sizes	Fat	Calories	Carbs	Protein
TOTALS						
Satisfied after eating?						

Meal 2		Portion Sizes	Fat	Calories	Carbs	Protein
TOTALS						
Satisfied after eating?						

Notes

Meal 3	Portion Sizes	Fat	Calories	Carbs	Protein
TOTALS					
Satisfied after eating?					

Meal 4	Portion Sizes	Fat	Calories	Carbs	Protein
TOTALS					
Satisfied after eating?					

Meal 5	Portion Sizes	Fat	Calories	Carbs	Protein
TOTALS					
Satisfied after eating?					

Daily Activity Log

Date/Time	Activity Description	How I Feel	Duration	Value

NOTES

Gratitude Journal

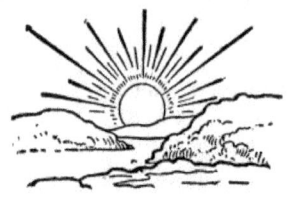

Today's been a Great Day
Because:_____

_____
_____
_____
_____
_____
_____
_____
_____
_____
_____
_____
_____
_____
_____
_____
_____
_____
_____
_____
_____
_____
_____

Example Affirmations you can use or use your own.

Goals:
>   I choose to set goals, and work to achieve them.
>   When I set a goal I reach and nothing can stop me.
>   I stay with my goals until accomplished.

Weight loss:
>   I live best when I eat less.
>   I eat only nourishing foods for my Mind, Body and soul.
>   I feel great at my perfect weight of 120 (fill in the weight you want to

weigh)

Self-Esteem:
>   I love myself more and more every day in every way.
>   I care about my wellbeing and take care of myself.
>   I love everything about me.

Exercise:
>   When I exercise I feel great.
>   I enjoy exercising
>   I choose to exercise regularly

Prosperity:
>   I am a money magnet and money flows freely to me.
>   Infinite riches are now freely flowing into my life.
>   It's okay for me to have everything I want.

Health:
>   I am healthier today and every day.
>   I choose to be healthy and it shows.
>   I am vibrantly healthy and radiantly beautiful.

Relationships:
>   I now give and receive love freely,
>   I am now attracting my perfect soul mate.
>   I love to love and be loved.

Happiness:
>   I feel happy and blissful every day.
>   Happiness follows me everywhere I go.
>   I only see and attract happiness.

Affirmations

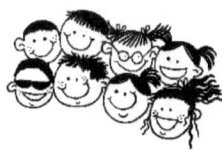

_____! (fill in your own affirmations)

_____

_____

_____

_____

_____

_____

_____

_____

_____

_____

_____

_____

_____

_____

_____

_____

_____

_____

_____

_____

_____

_____

_____

Date:_____

Day 15
To a New YOU!

Goal_____

_____

_____

_____

_____

_____

_____

_____

_____

What Makes your goal
specific?_____

_____

How can your goal be
measured?_____

_____

How is your goal
Attainable?_____

_____

What makes your goal
realistic?_____

_____

What is the timeline for your
goal?_____

_____

DAY #:＿＿＿＿＿＿

Meal 1	Portion Sizes	Fat	Calories	Carbs	Protein
TOTALS					
Satisfied after eating?					

Meal 2	Portion Sizes	Fat	Calories	Carbs	Protein
TOTALS					
Satisfied after eating?					

Notes

Meal 3	Portion Sizes	Fat	Calories	Carbs	Protein
TOTALS					
Satisfied after eating?					

Meal 4	Portion Sizes	Fat	Calories	Carbs	Protein
TOTALS					
Satisfied after eating?					

Meal 5	Portion Sizes	Fat	Calories	Carbs	Protein
TOTALS					
Satisfied after eating?					

Daily Activity Log

Date/Time	Activity Description	How I Feel	Duration	Value
NOTES				

Gratitude Journal

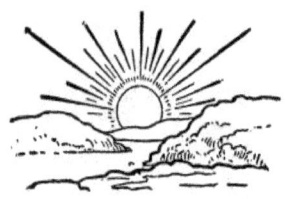

Today's been a Great Day
Because:_____

_____
_____
_____
_____
_____
_____
_____
_____
_____
_____
_____
_____
_____
_____
_____
_____
_____
_____
_____
_____
_____
_____
_____
_____
_____

Example Affirmations you can use or use your own.

Goals:

>   I choose to set goals, and work to achieve them.
>   When I set a goal I reach and nothing can stop me.
>   I stay with my goals until accomplished.

Weight loss:

>   I live best when I eat less.
>   I eat only nourishing foods for my Mind, Body and soul.
>   I feel great at my perfect weight of 120 (fill in the weight you want to

weigh)

Self-Esteem:

>   I love myself more and more every day in every way.
>   I care about my wellbeing and take care of myself.
>   I love everything about me.

Exercise:

>   When I exercise I feel great.
>   I enjoy exercising
>   I choose to exercise regularly

Prosperity:

>   I am a money magnet and money flows freely to me.
>   Infinite riches are now freely flowing into my life.
>   It's okay for me to have everything I want.

Health:

>   I am healthier today and every day.
>   I choose to be healthy and it shows.
>   I am vibrantly healthy and radiantly beautiful.

Relationships:

>   I now give and receive love freely,
>   I am now attracting my perfect soul mate.
>   I love to love and be loved.

Happiness:

>   I feel happy and blissful every day.
>   Happiness follows me everywhere I go.
>   I only see and attract happiness.

Affirmations

_____! (fill in your own affirmations)

_____

_____

_____

_____

_____

_____

_____

_____

_____

_____

_____

_____

_____

_____

_____

_____

_____

_____

_____

_____

_____

Date:_____

Day 16
To a New YOU!

Goal_____

_____

_____

_____

_____

_____

_____

_____

What Makes your goal
specific?_____

_____

How can your goal be
measured?_____

_____

How is your goal
Attainable?_____

_____

What makes your goal
realistic?_____

_____

What is the timeline for your
goal?_____

_____

DAY #:_____

Meal 1	Portion Sizes	Fat	Calories	Carbs	Protein
TOTALS					
Satisfied after eating?					

Meal 2	Portion Sizes	Fat	Calories	Carbs	Protein
TOTALS					
Satisfied after eating?					

Notes

Meal 3	Portion Sizes	Fat	Calories	Carbs	Protein
TOTALS					
Satisfied after eating?					

Meal 4	Portion Sizes	Fat	Calories	Carbs	Protein
TOTALS					
Satisfied after eating?					

Meal 5	Portion Sizes	Fat	Calories	Carbs	Protein
TOTALS					
Satisfied after eating?					

Daily Activity Log

Date/Time	Activity Description	How I Feel	Duration	Value
NOTES				

Gratitude Journal

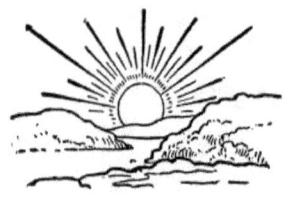

Today's been a Great Day
Because:_____

_____

_____

_____

_____

_____

_____

_____

_____

_____

_____

_____

_____

_____

_____

_____

_____

_____

_____

_____

_____

_____

_____

_____

Example Affirmations you can use or use your own.

Goals:

      I choose to set goals, and work to achieve them.

      When I set a goal I reach and nothing can stop me.

      I stay with my goals until accomplished.

Weight loss:

      I live best when I eat less.

      I eat only nourishing foods for my Mind, Body and soul.

      I feel great at my perfect weight of 120 (fill in the weight you want to weigh)

Self-Esteem:

      I love myself more and more every day in every way.

      I care about my wellbeing and take care of myself.

      I love everything about me.

Exercise:

      When I exercise I feel great.

      I enjoy exercising

      I choose to exercise regularly

Prosperity:

      I am a money magnet and money flows freely to me.

      Infinite riches are now freely flowing into my life.

      It's okay for me to have everything I want.

Health:

      I am healthier today and every day.

      I choose to be healthy and it shows.

      I am vibrantly healthy and radiantly beautiful.

Relationships:

      I now give and receive love freely,

      I am now attracting my perfect soul mate.

      I love to love and be loved.

Happiness:

      I feel happy and blissful every day.

      Happiness follows me everywhere I go.

      I only see and attract happiness.

Affirmations

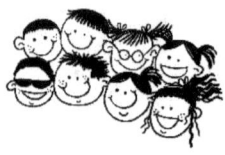

_____! (fill in your own affirmations)

_____

_____

_____

_____

_____

_____

_____

_____

_____

_____

_____

_____

_____

_____

_____

_____

_____

_____

_____

_____

_____

_____

_____

_____

_____

Date:_____

Day 17
To a New YOU!

Goal_____

_____

_____

_____

_____

_____

_____

_____

What Makes your goal specific?_____

_____

How can your goal be measured?_____

_____

How is your goal Attainable?_____

_____

What makes your goal realistic?_____

_____

What is the timeline for your goal?_____

_____

DAY #:_____

Meal 1	Portion Sizes	Fat	Calories	Carbs	Protein
TOTALS					
Satisfied after eating?					

Meal 2	Portion Sizes	Fat	Calories	Carbs	Protein
TOTALS					
Satisfied after eating?					

Notes

Meal 3	Portion Sizes	Fat	Calories	Carbs	Protein
TOTALS					
Satisfied after eating?					

Meal 4	Portion Sizes	Fat	Calories	Carbs	Protein
TOTALS					
Satisfied after eating?					

Meal 5	Portion Sizes	Fat	Calories	Carbs	Protein
TOTALS					
Satisfied after eating?					

Daily Activity Log

Date/Time	Activity Description	How I Feel	Duration	Value
NOTES				

Gratitude Journal

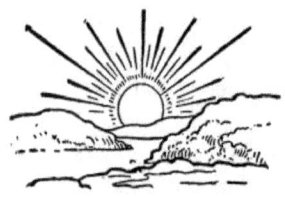

Today's been a Great Day
Because:_____

_____

_____

_____

_____

_____

_____

_____

_____

_____

_____

_____

_____

_____

_____

_____

_____

_____

_____

_____

_____

_____

_____

_____

Example Affirmations you can use or use your own.

Goals:

      I choose to set goals, and work to achieve them.

      When I set a goal I reach and nothing can stop me.

      I stay with my goals until accomplished.

Weight loss:

      I live best when I eat less.

      I eat only nourishing foods for my Mind, Body and soul.

      I feel great at my perfect weight of 120 (fill in the weight you want to weigh)

Self-Esteem:

      I love myself more and more every day in every way.

      I care about my wellbeing and take care of myself.

      I love everything about me.

Exercise:

      When I exercise I feel great.

      I enjoy exercising

      I choose to exercise regularly

Prosperity:

      I am a money magnet and money flows freely to me.

      Infinite riches are now freely flowing into my life.

      It's okay for me to have everything I want.

Health:

      I am healthier today and every day.

      I choose to be healthy and it shows.

      I am vibrantly healthy and radiantly beautiful.

Relationships:

      I now give and receive love freely,

      I am now attracting my perfect soul mate.

      I love to love and be loved.

Happiness:

      I feel happy and blissful every day.

      Happiness follows me everywhere I go.

      I only see and attract happiness.

Affirmations

_____! (fill in your own affirmations)

_____

_____

_____

_____

_____

_____

_____

_____

_____

_____

_____

_____

_____

_____

_____

_____

_____

_____

_____

_____

_____

_____

_____

Date:_____

Day 18
To a New YOU!

Goal_____

_____

_____

_____

_____

_____

_____

_____

What Makes your goal
specific?_____

_____

How can your goal be
measured?_____

_____

How is your goal
Attainable?_____

_____

What makes your goal
realistic?_____

_____

What is the timeline for your
goal?_____

_____

DAY #:_____

Meal 1	Portion Sizes	Fat	Calories	Carbs	Protein
TOTALS					
Satisfied after eating?					

Meal 2	Portion Sizes	Fat	Calories	Carbs	Protein
TOTALS					
Satisfied after eating?					

Notes

Meal 3	Portion Sizes	Fat	Calories	Carbs	Protein
TOTALS					
Satisfied after eating?					

Meal 4	Portion Sizes	Fat	Calories	Carbs	Protein
TOTALS					
Satisfied after eating?					

Meal 5	Portion Sizes	Fat	Calories	Carbs	Protein
TOTALS					
Satisfied after eating?					

Daily Activity Log

Date/Time	Activity Description	How I Feel	Duration	Value
NOTES				

Gratitude Journal

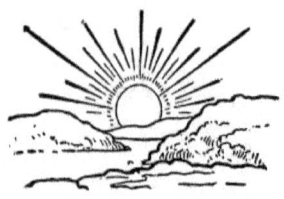

Today's been a Great Day
Because:_____

_____

_____

_____

_____

_____

_____

_____

_____

_____

_____

_____

_____

_____

_____

_____

_____

_____

_____

_____

_____

_____

_____

_____

_____

_____

Example Affirmations you can use or use your own.

Goals:

I choose to set goals, and work to achieve them.

When I set a goal I reach and nothing can stop me.

I stay with my goals until accomplished.

Weight loss:

I live best when I eat less.

I eat only nourishing foods for my Mind, Body and soul.

I feel great at my perfect weight of 120 (fill in the weight you want to weigh)

Self-Esteem:

I love myself more and more every day in every way.

I care about my wellbeing and take care of myself.

I love everything about me.

Exercise:

When I exercise I feel great.

I enjoy exercising

I choose to exercise regularly

Prosperity:

I am a money magnet and money flows freely to me.

Infinite riches are now freely flowing into my life.

It's okay for me to have everything I want.

Health:

I am healthier today and every day.

I choose to be healthy and it shows.

I am vibrantly healthy and radiantly beautiful.

Relationships:

I now give and receive love freely,

I am now attracting my perfect soul mate.

I love to love and be loved.

Happiness:

I feel happy and blissful every day.

Happiness follows me everywhere I go.

I only see and attract happiness.

Affirmations

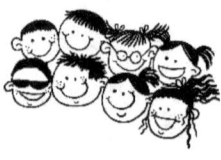

_____! (fill in your own affirmations)

_____

_____

_____

_____

_____

_____

_____

_____

_____

_____

_____

_____

_____

_____

_____

_____

_____

_____

_____

_____

_____

_____

_____

_____

Date:_____

Day 19
To a New YOU!

Goal_____

_____

_____

_____

_____

_____

_____

_____

What Makes your goal
specific?_____

_____

How can your goal be
measured?_____

_____

How is your goal
Attainable?_____

_____

What makes your goal
realistic?_____

_____

What is the timeline for your
goal?_____

_____

DAY #:_____

Meal 1	Portion Sizes	Fat	Calories	Carbs	Protein
TOTALS					
Satisfied after eating?					

Meal 2	Portion Sizes	Fat	Calories	Carbs	Protein
TOTALS					
Satisfied after eating?					

Notes

Meal 3	Portion Sizes	Fat	Calories	Carbs	Protein
TOTALS					
Satisfied after eating?					

Meal 4	Portion Sizes	Fat	Calories	Carbs	Protein
TOTALS					
Satisfied after eating?					

Meal 5	Portion Sizes	Fat	Calories	Carbs	Protein
TOTALS					
Satisfied after eating?					

Daily Activity Log

Date/Time	Activity Description	How I Feel	Duration	Value
NOTES				

Gratitude Journal

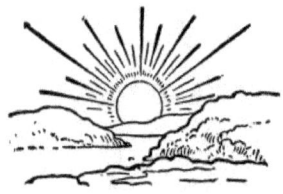

Today's been a Great Day
Because:_____

_____
_____
_____
_____
_____
_____
_____
_____
_____
_____
_____
_____
_____
_____
_____
_____
_____
_____
_____
_____
_____
_____

Example Affirmations you can use or use your own.

Goals:

> I choose to set goals, and work to achieve them.
> When I set a goal I reach and nothing can stop me.
> I stay with my goals until accomplished.

Weight loss:

> I live best when I eat less.
> I eat only nourishing foods for my Mind, Body and soul.
> I feel great at my perfect weight of 120 (fill in the weight you want to weigh)

Self-Esteem:

> I love myself more and more every day in every way.
> I care about my wellbeing and take care of myself.
> I love everything about me.

Exercise:

> When I exercise I feel great.
> I enjoy exercising
> I choose to exercise regularly

Prosperity:

> I am a money magnet and money flows freely to me.
> Infinite riches are now freely flowing into my life.
> It's okay for me to have everything I want.

Health:

> I am healthier today and every day.
> I choose to be healthy and it shows.
> I am vibrantly healthy and radiantly beautiful.

Relationships:

> I now give and receive love freely,
> I am now attracting my perfect soul mate.
> I love to love and be loved.

Happiness:

> I feel happy and blissful every day.
> Happiness follows me everywhere I go.
> I only see and attract happiness.

Affirmations

_____! (fill in your own affirmations)

_____

_____

_____

_____

_____

_____

_____

_____

_____

_____

_____

_____

_____

_____

_____

_____

_____

_____

_____

_____

_____

_____

_____

_____

_____

Date:_____

Day 20
To a New YOU!

Goal_____

_____

_____

_____

_____

_____

_____

_____

What Makes your goal
specific?_____
_____

How can your goal be
measured?_____
_____

How is your goal
Attainable?_____
_____

What makes your goal
realistic?_____
_____

What is the timeline for your
goal?_____
_____

DAY #:_____

Meal 1	Portion Sizes	Fat	Calories	Carbs	Protein
TOTALS					
Satisfied after eating?					

Meal 2	Portion Sizes	Fat	Calories	Carbs	Protein
TOTALS					
Satisfied after eating?					

Notes

Meal 3	Portion Sizes	Fat	Calories	Carbs	Protein
TOTALS					
Satisfied after eating?					

Meal 4	Portion Sizes	Fat	Calories	Carbs	Protein
TOTALS					
Satisfied after eating?					

Meal 5	Portion Sizes	Fat	Calories	Carbs	Protein
TOTALS					
Satisfied after eating?					

Daily Activity Log

Date/Time	Activity Description	How I Feel	Duration	Value
NOTES				

Gratitude Journal

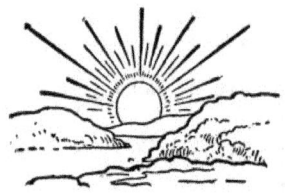

Today's been a Great Day
Because:_____

_____
_____
_____
_____
_____
_____
_____
_____
_____
_____
_____
_____
_____
_____
_____
_____
_____
_____
_____
_____
_____
_____
_____
_____

Example Affirmations you can use or use your own.

Goals:

      I choose to set goals, and work to achieve them.

      When I set a goal I reach and nothing can stop me.

      I stay with my goals until accomplished.

Weight loss:

      I live best when I eat less.

      I eat only nourishing foods for my Mind, Body and soul.

      I feel great at my perfect weight of 120 (fill in the weight you want to weigh)

Self-Esteem:

      I love myself more and more every day in every way.

      I care about my wellbeing and take care of myself.

      I love everything about me.

Exercise:

      When I exercise I feel great.

      I enjoy exercising

      I choose to exercise regularly

Prosperity:

      I am a money magnet and money flows freely to me.

      Infinite riches are now freely flowing into my life.

      It's okay for me to have everything I want.

Health:

      I am healthier today and every day.

      I choose to be healthy and it shows.

      I am vibrantly healthy and radiantly beautiful.

Relationships:

      I now give and receive love freely,

      I am now attracting my perfect soul mate.

      I love to love and be loved.

Happiness:

      I feel happy and blissful every day.

      Happiness follows me everywhere I go.

      I only see and attract happiness.

Affirmations

_____! (fill in your own affirmations)

_____

_____

_____

_____

_____

_____

_____

_____

_____

_____

_____

_____

_____

_____

_____

_____

_____

_____

_____

_____

_____

_____

_____

Date:_____

Day 21
To a New YOU!

Goal_____

_____

_____

_____

_____

_____

_____

_____

What Makes your goal
specific?_____

_____

How can your goal be
measured?_____

_____

How is your goal
Attainable?_____

_____

What makes your goal
realistic?_____

_____

What is the timeline for your
goal?_____

_____

DAY #:_____

Meal 1	Portion Sizes	Fat	Calories	Carbs	Protein
TOTALS					
Satisfied after eating?					

Meal 2	Portion Sizes	Fat	Calories	Carbs	Protein
TOTALS					
Satisfied after eating?					

Notes

Meal 3	Portion Sizes	Fat	Calories	Carbs	Protein
TOTALS					
Satisfied after eating?					

Meal 4	Portion Sizes	Fat	Calories	Carbs	Protein
TOTALS					
Satisfied after eating?					

Meal 5	Portion Sizes	Fat	Calories	Carbs	Protein
TOTALS					
Satisfied after eating?					

Daily Activity Log

Date/Time	Activity Description	How I Feel	Duration	Value
NOTES				

Gratitude Journal

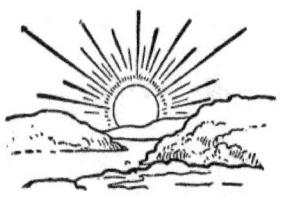

Today's been a Great Day
Because:_____

_____
_____
_____
_____
_____
_____
_____
_____
_____
_____
_____
_____
_____
_____
_____
_____
_____
_____
_____
_____
_____
_____

Example Affirmations you can use or use your own.

Goals:

> I choose to set goals, and work to achieve them.
> When I set a goal I reach and nothing can stop me.
> I stay with my goals until accomplished.

Weight loss:

> I live best when I eat less.
> I eat only nourishing foods for my Mind, Body and soul.
> I feel great at my perfect weight of 120 (fill in the weight you want to weigh)

Self-Esteem:

> I love myself more and more every day in every way.
> I care about my wellbeing and take care of myself.
> I love everything about me.

Exercise:

> When I exercise I feel great.
> I enjoy exercising
> I choose to exercise regularly

Prosperity:

> I am a money magnet and money flows freely to me.
> Infinite riches are now freely flowing into my life.
> It's okay for me to have everything I want.

Health:

> I am healthier today and every day.
> I choose to be healthy and it shows.
> I am vibrantly healthy and radiantly beautiful.

Relationships:

> I now give and receive love freely,
> I am now attracting my perfect soul mate.
> I love to love and be loved.

Happiness:

> I feel happy and blissful every day.
> Happiness follows me everywhere I go.
> I only see and attract happiness.

Affirmations

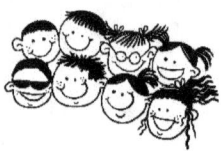

_____! (fill in your own affirmations)

_____

_____

_____

_____

_____

_____

_____

_____

_____

_____

_____

_____

_____

_____

_____

_____

_____

_____

_____

_____

_____

_____

_____

Date:_____

Day 22
To a New YOU!

Goal_____

_____

_____

_____

_____

_____

_____

_____

_____

What Makes your goal
specific?_____

_____

How can your goal be
measured?_____

_____

How is your goal
Attainable?_____

_____

What makes your goal
realistic?_____

_____

What is the timeline for your
goal?_____

_____

DAY #:_____

Meal 1	Portion Sizes	Fat	Calories	Carbs	Protein
TOTALS					
Satisfied after eating?					

Meal 2	Portion Sizes	Fat	Calories	Carbs	Protein
TOTALS					
Satisfied after eating?					

Notes

Meal 3	Portion Sizes	Fat	Calories	Carbs	Protein
TOTALS					
Satisfied after eating?					

Meal 4	Portion Sizes	Fat	Calories	Carbs	Protein
TOTALS					
Satisfied after eating?					

Meal 5	Portion Sizes	Fat	Calories	Carbs	Protein
TOTALS					
Satisfied after eating?					

Daily Activity Log

Date/Time	Activity Description	How I Feel	Duration	Value
NOTES				

Gratitude Journal

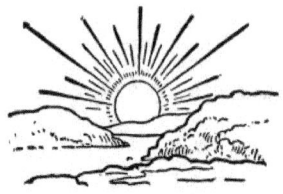

Today's been a Great Day
Because:_____

_____
_____
_____
_____
_____
_____
_____
_____
_____
_____
_____
_____
_____
_____
_____
_____
_____
_____
_____
_____
_____
_____
_____
_____

Example Affirmations you can use or use your own.

Goals:

>I choose to set goals, and work to achieve them.
>When I set a goal I reach and nothing can stop me.
>I stay with my goals until accomplished.

Weight loss:

>I live best when I eat less.
>I eat only nourishing foods for my Mind, Body and soul.
>I feel great at my perfect weight of 120 (fill in the weight you want to weigh)

Self-Esteem:

>I love myself more and more every day in every way.
>I care about my wellbeing and take care of myself.
>I love everything about me.

Exercise:

>When I exercise I feel great.
>I enjoy exercising
>I choose to exercise regularly

Prosperity:

>I am a money magnet and money flows freely to me.
>Infinite riches are now freely flowing into my life.
>It's okay for me to have everything I want.

Health:

>I am healthier today and every day.
>I choose to be healthy and it shows.
>I am vibrantly healthy and radiantly beautiful.

Relationships:

>I now give and receive love freely,
>I am now attracting my perfect soul mate.
>I love to love and be loved.

Happiness:

>I feel happy and blissful every day.
>Happiness follows me everywhere I go.
>I only see and attract happiness.

Affirmations

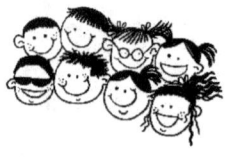

_____! (fill in your own affirmations)

_____

_____

_____

_____

_____

_____

_____

_____

_____

_____

_____

_____

_____

_____

_____

_____

_____

_____

_____

_____

_____

_____

_____

Date:_____

Day 23
To a New YOU!

Goal_____

_____

_____

_____

_____

_____

_____

_____

What Makes your goal
specific?_____

_____

How can your goal be
measured?_____

_____

How is your goal
Attainable?_____

_____

What makes your goal
realistic?_____

_____

What is the timeline for your
goal?_____

_____

DAY #:_____

Meal 1	Portion Sizes	Fat	Calories	Carbs	Protein
TOTALS					
Satisfied after eating?					

Meal 2	Portion Sizes	Fat	Calories	Carbs	Protein
TOTALS					
Satisfied after eating?					

Notes

Meal 3	Portion Sizes	Fat	Calories	Carbs	Protein
TOTALS					
Satisfied after eating?					

Meal 4	Portion Sizes	Fat	Calories	Carbs	Protein
TOTALS					
Satisfied after eating?					

Meal 5	Portion Sizes	Fat	Calories	Carbs	Protein
TOTALS					
Satisfied after eating?					

Daily Activity Log

Date/Time	Activity Description	How I Feel	Duration	Value
NOTES				

Gratitude Journal

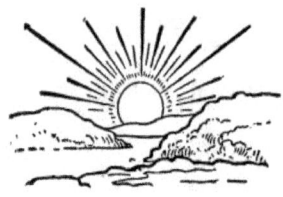

Today's been a Great Day
Because:_____

_____

_____

_____

_____

_____

_____

_____

_____

_____

_____

_____

_____

_____

_____

_____

_____

_____

_____

_____

_____

_____

_____

_____

_____

_____

_____

_____

Example Affirmations you can use or use your own.

Goals:
> I choose to set goals, and work to achieve them.
> When I set a goal I reach and nothing can stop me.
> I stay with my goals until accomplished.

Weight loss:
> I live best when I eat less.
> I eat only nourishing foods for my Mind, Body and soul.
> I feel great at my perfect weight of 120 (fill in the weight you want to weigh)

Self-Esteem:
> I love myself more and more every day in every way.
> I care about my wellbeing and take care of myself.
> I love everything about me.

Exercise:
> When I exercise I feel great.
> I enjoy exercising
> I choose to exercise regularly

Prosperity:
> I am a money magnet and money flows freely to me.
> Infinite riches are now freely flowing into my life.
> It's okay for me to have everything I want.

Health:
> I am healthier today and every day.
> I choose to be healthy and it shows.
> I am vibrantly healthy and radiantly beautiful.

Relationships:
> I now give and receive love freely,
> I am now attracting my perfect soul mate.
> I love to love and be loved.

Happiness:
> I feel happy and blissful every day.
> Happiness follows me everywhere I go.
> I only see and attract happiness.

Affirmations

_____! (fill in your own affirmations)

Date:_____

Day 24
To a New YOU!

Goal_____

_____

_____

_____

_____

_____

_____

_____

What Makes your goal
specific?_____

_____

How can your goal be
measured?_____

_____

How is your goal
Attainable?_____

_____

What makes your goal
realistic?_____

_____

What is the timeline for your
goal?_____

_____

DAY #:_____

Meal 1	Portion Sizes	Fat	Calories	Carbs	Protein
TOTALS					
Satisfied after eating?					

Meal 2	Portion Sizes	Fat	Calories	Carbs	Protein
TOTALS					
Satisfied after eating?					

Notes

Meal 3	Portion Sizes	Fat	Calories	Carbs	Protein
TOTALS					
Satisfied after eating?					

Meal 4	Portion Sizes	Fat	Calories	Carbs	Protein
TOTALS					
Satisfied after eating?					

Meal 5	Portion Sizes	Fat	Calories	Carbs	Protein
TOTALS					
Satisfied after eating?					

Daily Activity Log

Date/Time	Activity Description	How I Feel	Duration	Value
NOTES				

Gratitude Journal

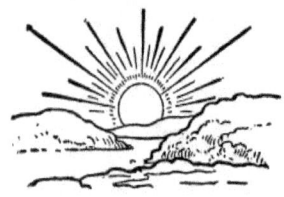

Today's been a Great Day
Because:_____

_____

_____
_____
_____
_____
_____
_____
_____
_____
_____
_____
_____
_____
_____
_____
_____
_____
_____
_____
_____
_____
_____
_____
_____
_____
_____
_____

Example Affirmations you can use or use your own.

Goals:

> I choose to set goals, and work to achieve them.
> When I set a goal I reach and nothing can stop me.
> I stay with my goals until accomplished.

Weight loss:

> I live best when I eat less.
> I eat only nourishing foods for my Mind, Body and soul.
> I feel great at my perfect weight of 120 (fill in the weight you want to weigh)

Self-Esteem:

> I love myself more and more every day in every way.
> I care about my wellbeing and take care of myself.
> I love everything about me.

Exercise:

> When I exercise I feel great.
> I enjoy exercising
> I choose to exercise regularly

Prosperity:

> I am a money magnet and money flows freely to me.
> Infinite riches are now freely flowing into my life.
> It's okay for me to have everything I want.

Health:

> I am healthier today and every day.
> I choose to be healthy and it shows.
> I am vibrantly healthy and radiantly beautiful.

Relationships:

> I now give and receive love freely,
> I am now attracting my perfect soul mate.
> I love to love and be loved.

Happiness:

> I feel happy and blissful every day.
> Happiness follows me everywhere I go.
> I only see and attract happiness.

Affirmations

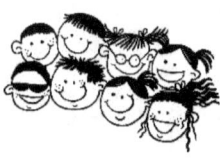

_____! (fill in your own affirmations)

_____

_____

_____

_____

_____

_____

_____

_____

_____

_____

_____

_____

_____

_____

_____

_____

_____

_____

_____

_____

_____

_____

Date:_____

Day 25
To a New YOU!

Goal_____

_____

_____

_____

_____

_____

_____

_____

What Makes your goal
specific?_____

_____

How can your goal be
measured?_____

_____

How is your goal
Attainable?_____

_____

What makes your goal
realistic?_____

_____

What is the timeline for your
goal?_____

_____

DAY #: _____

Meal 1	Portion Sizes	Fat	Calories	Carbs	Protein
TOTALS					
Satisfied after eating?					

Meal 2	Portion Sizes	Fat	Calories	Carbs	Protein
TOTALS					
Satisfied after eating?					

Notes

Meal 3	Portion Sizes	Fat	Calories	Carbs	Protein
TOTALS					
Satisfied after eating?					

Meal 4	Portion Sizes	Fat	Calories	Carbs	Protein
TOTALS					
Satisfied after eating?					

Meal 5	Portion Sizes	Fat	Calories	Carbs	Protein
TOTALS					
Satisfied after eating?					

Daily Activity Log

Date/Time	Activity Description	How I Feel	Duration	Value
NOTES				

Gratitude Journal

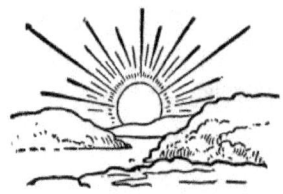

Today's been a Great Day
Because:_____

_____
_____
_____
_____
_____
_____
_____
_____
_____
_____
_____
_____
_____
_____
_____
_____
_____
_____
_____
_____
_____

Example Affirmations you can use or use your own.

Goals:
>   I choose to set goals, and work to achieve them.
>   When I set a goal I reach and nothing can stop me.
>   I stay with my goals until accomplished.

Weight loss:
>   I live best when I eat less.
>   I eat only nourishing foods for my Mind, Body and soul.
>   I feel great at my perfect weight of 120 (fill in the weight you want to
weigh)

Self-Esteem:
>   I love myself more and more every day in every way.
>   I care about my wellbeing and take care of myself.
>   I love everything about me.

Exercise:
>   When I exercise I feel great.
>   I enjoy exercising
>   I choose to exercise regularly

Prosperity:
>   I am a money magnet and money flows freely to me.
>   Infinite riches are now freely flowing into my life.
>   It's okay for me to have everything I want.

Health:
>   I am healthier today and every day.
>   I choose to be healthy and it shows.
>   I am vibrantly healthy and radiantly beautiful.

Relationships:
>   I now give and receive love freely,
>   I am now attracting my perfect soul mate.
>   I love to love and be loved.

Happiness:
>   I feel happy and blissful every day.
>   Happiness follows me everywhere I go.
>   I only see and attract happiness.

Affirmations

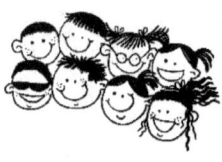

_____! (fill in your own affirmations)

_____

_____

_____

_____

_____

_____

_____

_____

_____

_____

_____

_____

_____

_____

_____

_____

_____

_____

_____

_____

_____

_____

_____

Date:_____

Day 26
To a New YOU!

Goal_____

_____

_____

_____

_____

_____

_____

_____

What Makes your goal specific?_____

_____

How can your goal be measured?_____

_____

How is your goal Attainable?_____

_____

What makes your goal realistic?_____

_____

What is the timeline for your goal?_____

_____

DAY #:_____

Meal 1	Portion Sizes	Fat	Calories	Carbs	Protein
TOTALS					
Satisfied after eating?					

Meal 2	Portion Sizes	Fat	Calories	Carbs	Protein
TOTALS					
Satisfied after eating?					

Notes

Meal 3	Portion Sizes	Fat	Calories	Carbs	Protein
TOTALS					
Satisfied after eating?					

Meal 4	Portion Sizes	Fat	Calories	Carbs	Protein
TOTALS					
Satisfied after eating?					

Meal 5	Portion Sizes	Fat	Calories	Carbs	Protein
TOTALS					
Satisfied after eating?					

Daily Activity Log

Date/Time	Activity Description	How I Feel	Duration	Value
NOTES				

Gratitude Journal

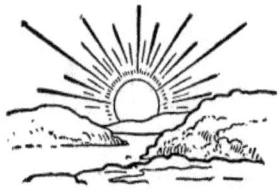

Today's been a Great Day
Because:_____

_____
_____
_____
_____
_____
_____
_____
_____
_____
_____
_____
_____
_____
_____
_____
_____
_____
_____
_____
_____
_____
_____
_____

Example Affirmations you can use or use your own.

Goals:

I choose to set goals, and work to achieve them.

When I set a goal I reach and nothing can stop me.

I stay with my goals until accomplished.

Weight loss:

I live best when I eat less.

I eat only nourishing foods for my Mind, Body and soul.

I feel great at my perfect weight of 120 (fill in the weight you want to weigh)

Self-Esteem:

I love myself more and more every day in every way.

I care about my wellbeing and take care of myself.

I love everything about me.

Exercise:

When I exercise I feel great.

I enjoy exercising

I choose to exercise regularly

Prosperity:

I am a money magnet and money flows freely to me.

Infinite riches are now freely flowing into my life.

It's okay for me to have everything I want.

Health:

I am healthier today and every day.

I choose to be healthy and it shows.

I am vibrantly healthy and radiantly beautiful.

Relationships:

I now give and receive love freely,

I am now attracting my perfect soul mate.

I love to love and be loved.

Happiness:

I feel happy and blissful every day.

Happiness follows me everywhere I go.

I only see and attract happiness.

Affirmations

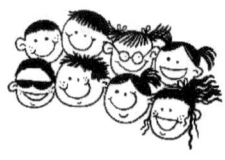

_____! (fill in your own affirmations)

_____

_____

_____

_____

_____

_____

_____

_____

_____

_____

_____

_____

_____

_____

_____

_____

_____

_____

_____

_____

_____

Date:_____

Day 27
To a New YOU!

Goal_____

_____

_____

_____

_____

_____

_____

_____

_____

What Makes your goal
specific?_____

_____

How can your goal be
measured?_____

_____

How is your goal
Attainable?_____

_____

What makes your goal
realistic?_____

_____

What is the timeline for your
goal?_____

_____

DAY #:_____

Meal 1	Portion Sizes	Fat	Calories	Carbs	Protein
TOTALS					
Satisfied after eating?					

Meal 2	Portion Sizes	Fat	Calories	Carbs	Protein
TOTALS					
Satisfied after eating?					

Notes

Meal 3	Portion Sizes	Fat	Calories	Carbs	Protein
TOTALS					
Satisfied after eating?					

Meal 4	Portion Sizes	Fat	Calories	Carbs	Protein
TOTALS					
Satisfied after eating?					

Meal 5	Portion Sizes	Fat	Calories	Carbs	Protein
TOTALS					
Satisfied after eating?					

Daily Activity Log

Date/Time	Activity Description	How I Feel	Duration	Value
NOTES				

Gratitude Journal

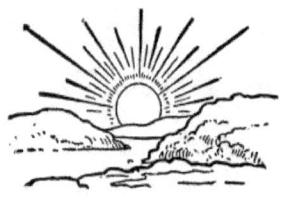

Today's been a Great Day
Because:_____

_____
_____
_____
_____
_____
_____
_____
_____
_____
_____
_____
_____
_____
_____
_____
_____
_____
_____
_____
_____
_____
_____
_____

Example Affirmations you can use or use your own.

Goals:

>I choose to set goals, and work to achieve them.
>When I set a goal I reach and nothing can stop me.
>I stay with my goals until accomplished.

Weight loss:

>I live best when I eat less.
>I eat only nourishing foods for my Mind, Body and soul.
>I feel great at my perfect weight of 120 (fill in the weight you want to

weigh)

Self-Esteem:

>I love myself more and more every day in every way.
>I care about my wellbeing and take care of myself.
>I love everything about me.

Exercise:

>When I exercise I feel great.
>I enjoy exercising
>I choose to exercise regularly

Prosperity:

>I am a money magnet and money flows freely to me.
>Infinite riches are now freely flowing into my life.
>It's okay for me to have everything I want.

Health:

>I am healthier today and every day.
>I choose to be healthy and it shows.
>I am vibrantly healthy and radiantly beautiful.

Relationships:

>I now give and receive love freely,
>I am now attracting my perfect soul mate.
>I love to love and be loved.

Happiness:

>I feel happy and blissful every day.
>Happiness follows me everywhere I go.
>I only see and attract happiness.

Affirmations

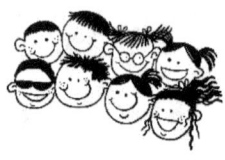

_____! (fill in your own affirmations)

_____

_____

_____

_____

_____

_____

_____

_____

_____

_____

_____

_____

_____

_____

_____

_____

_____

_____

_____

_____

_____

Date:_____

Day 28
To a New YOU!

Goal_____

_____

_____

_____

_____

_____

_____

_____

What Makes your goal specific?_____

_____

How can your goal be measured?_____

_____

How is your goal Attainable?_____

_____

What makes your goal realistic?_____

_____

What is the timeline for your goal?_____

_____

DAY #:_____

Meal 1	Portion Sizes	Fat	Calories	Carbs	Protein
TOTALS					
Satisfied after eating?					

Meal 2	Portion Sizes	Fat	Calories	Carbs	Protein
TOTALS					
Satisfied after eating?					

Notes

Meal 3	Portion Sizes	Fat	Calories	Carbs	Protein
TOTALS					
Satisfied after eating?					

Meal 4	Portion Sizes	Fat	Calories	Carbs	Protein
TOTALS					
Satisfied after eating?					

Meal 5	Portion Sizes	Fat	Calories	Carbs	Protein
TOTALS					
Satisfied after eating?					

Daily Activity Log

Date/Time	Activity Description	How I Feel	Duration	Value
NOTES				

Gratitude Journal

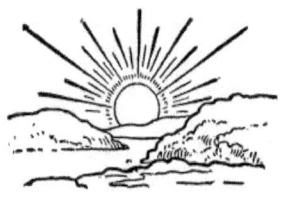

Today's been a Great Day
Because:_____

_____

_____

_____

_____

_____

_____

_____

_____

_____

_____

_____

_____

_____

_____

_____

_____

_____

_____

_____

_____

_____

_____

_____

Example Affirmations you can use or use your own.

Goals:

     I choose to set goals, and work to achieve them.

     When I set a goal I reach and nothing can stop me.

     I stay with my goals until accomplished.

Weight loss:

     I live best when I eat less.

     I eat only nourishing foods for my Mind, Body and soul.

     I feel great at my perfect weight of 120 (fill in the weight you want to weigh)

Self-Esteem:

     I love myself more and more every day in every way.

     I care about my wellbeing and take care of myself.

     I love everything about me.

Exercise:

     When I exercise I feel great.

     I enjoy exercising

     I choose to exercise regularly

Prosperity:

     I am a money magnet and money flows freely to me.

     Infinite riches are now freely flowing into my life.

     It's okay for me to have everything I want.

Health:

     I am healthier today and every day.

     I choose to be healthy and it shows.

     I am vibrantly healthy and radiantly beautiful.

Relationships:

     I now give and receive love freely,

     I am now attracting my perfect soul mate.

     I love to love and be loved.

Happiness:

     I feel happy and blissful every day.

     Happiness follows me everywhere I go.

     I only see and attract happiness.

Affirmations

_____! (fill in your own affirmations)

_____

_____

_____

_____

_____

_____

_____

_____

_____

_____

_____

_____

_____

_____

_____

_____

_____

_____

_____

_____

_____

_____

_____

_____

_____

Date:_____

Day 29
To a New YOU!

Goal_____

_____

_____

_____

_____

_____

_____

_____

_____

What Makes your goal
specific?_____
_____

How can your goal be
measured?_____
_____

How is your goal
Attainable?_____
_____

What makes your goal
realistic?_____
_____

What is the timeline for your
goal?_____
_____

DAY #:_____

Meal 1	Portion Sizes	Fat	Calories	Carbs	Protein
TOTALS					
Satisfied after eating?					

Meal 2	Portion Sizes	Fat	Calories	Carbs	Protein
TOTALS					
Satisfied after eating?					

Notes

Meal 3	Portion Sizes	Fat	Calories	Carbs	Protein
TOTALS					
Satisfied after eating?					

Meal 4	Portion Sizes	Fat	Calories	Carbs	Protein
TOTALS					
Satisfied after eating?					

Meal 5	Portion Sizes	Fat	Calories	Carbs	Protein
TOTALS					
Satisfied after eating?					

Daily Activity Log

Date/Time	Activity Description	How I Feel	Duration	Value
NOTES				

Gratitude Journal

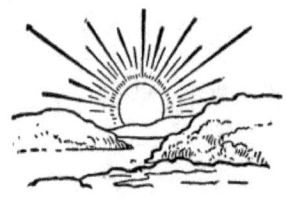

Today's been a Great Day
Because:_____

_____

_____

_____

_____

_____

_____

_____

_____

_____

_____

_____

_____

_____

_____

_____

_____

_____

_____

_____

_____

_____

_____

_____

_____

_____

_____

_____

_____

_____

_____

_____

Example Affirmations you can use or use your own.

Goals:

> I choose to set goals, and work to achieve them.
> When I set a goal I reach and nothing can stop me.
> I stay with my goals until accomplished.

Weight loss:

> I live best when I eat less.
> I eat only nourishing foods for my Mind, Body and soul.
> I feel great at my perfect weight of 120 (fill in the weight you want to weigh)

Self-Esteem:

> I love myself more and more every day in every way.
> I care about my wellbeing and take care of myself.
> I love everything about me.

Exercise:

> When I exercise I feel great.
> I enjoy exercising
> I choose to exercise regularly

Prosperity:

> I am a money magnet and money flows freely to me.
> Infinite riches are now freely flowing into my life.
> It's okay for me to have everything I want.

Health:

> I am healthier today and every day.
> I choose to be healthy and it shows.
> I am vibrantly healthy and radiantly beautiful.

Relationships:

> I now give and receive love freely,
> I am now attracting my perfect soul mate.
> I love to love and be loved.

Happiness:

> I feel happy and blissful every day.
> Happiness follows me everywhere I go.
> I only see and attract happiness.

Affirmations

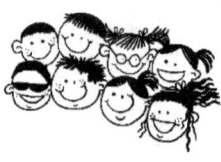

_____! (fill in your own affirmations)

_____

_____

_____

_____

_____

_____

_____

_____

_____

_____

_____

_____

_____

_____

_____

_____

_____

_____

_____

_____

_____

_____

_____

Date:_____

Day 30
To a New YOU!

Goal_____

_____

_____

_____

_____

_____

_____

_____

What Makes your goal
specific?_____

_____

How can your goal be
measured?_____

_____

How is your goal
Attainable?_____

_____

What makes your goal
realistic?_____

_____

What is the timeline for your
goal?_____

_____

DAY #:_____

Meal 1	Portion Sizes	Fat	Calories	Carbs	Protein
TOTALS					
Satisfied after eating?					

Meal 2	Portion Sizes	Fat	Calories	Carbs	Protein
TOTALS					
Satisfied after eating?					

Notes

Meal 3	Portion Sizes	Fat	Calories	Carbs	Protein
TOTALS					
Satisfied after eating?					

Meal 4	Portion Sizes	Fat	Calories	Carbs	Protein
TOTALS					
Satisfied after eating?					

Meal 5	Portion Sizes	Fat	Calories	Carbs	Protein
TOTALS					
Satisfied after eating?					

Daily Activity Log

Date/Time	Activity Description	How I Feel	Duration	Value
NOTES				

Gratitude Journal

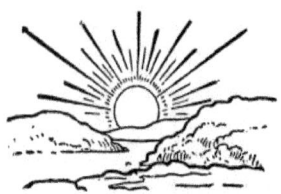

Today's been a Great Day
Because:_____

_____
_____
_____
_____
_____
_____
_____
_____
_____
_____
_____
_____
_____
_____
_____
_____
_____
_____
_____
_____
_____
_____
_____
_____
_____

Example Affirmations you can use or use your own.

Goals:

     I choose to set goals, and work to achieve them.

     When I set a goal I reach and nothing can stop me.

     I stay with my goals until accomplished.

Weight loss:

     I live best when I eat less.

     I eat only nourishing foods for my Mind, Body and soul.

     I feel great at my perfect weight of 120 (fill in the weight you want to

weigh)

Self-Esteem:

     I love myself more and more every day in every way.

     I care about my wellbeing and take care of myself.

     I love everything about me.

Exercise:

     When I exercise I feel great.

     I enjoy exercising

     I choose to exercise regularly

Prosperity:

     I am a money magnet and money flows freely to me.

     Infinite riches are now freely flowing into my life.

     It's okay for me to have everything I want.

Health:

     I am healthier today and every day.

     I choose to be healthy and it shows.

     I am vibrantly healthy and radiantly beautiful.

Relationships:

     I now give and receive love freely,

     I am now attracting my perfect soul mate.

     I love to love and be loved.

Happiness:

     I feel happy and blissful every day.

     Happiness follows me everywhere I go.

     I only see and attract happiness.

Affirmations

_____! (fill in your own affirmations)

About Cristie

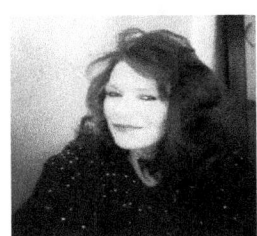

Cristie was born and raised in Hobbs, New Mexico. She moved to Colorado 18 years ago and still living there loving all the beauty Colorado has to offer. She has a daughter Lauren and a son Josh along with beautiful grandchildren. She has been an accountant the last 30 years. Not only an accountant and Health Coach but a teacher as well, teaching QuickBooks, cooking, detoxing and weight loss classes too!

In 2012, she lost her husband to lung cancer. After losing her husband to lung cancer she needed to make changes in her own health, so she did. Cristie went through a life transformation losing 200 pounds and went back to school to become a Nutritional Heath Coach adding Cleansing Intensive certification. She obtained her education from Institute of Integrative Nutrition for her Health Coaching. Her education for the Cleansing Intensive education was under Dr. Terry Willard CIH, PHD at the Wild Rose College. She is currently studying to add FDN, Functional Diagnostic Nutritionist to her skills to be able to help even more people.

Besides helping others, Cristie's other passion is to write. She has written 5 cookbooks, 2 of them are political collector's cookbooks. She didn't stop with cookbooks she also wrote "Veteran's Day Chase, a CIA political thriller, along with a QuickBooks Step by Step Guide. She has written 4 health and weight loss books. Last but not least she published a Car buying guide that her late husband had written with his vast knowledge and experience in the car industry.